Contents

Foreword 2

Welcome to the Food & M...

Food & mood and you 4

Changing what you eat 5

Keeping a food & mood diary 6

The stressors of life 7

Recipe 8

Sugar
  Quiz: am I sugar sensitive? 9
  Is sugar sensitivity a problem? 10
  How to manage sugar sensitivity 11

Caffeine
  Quiz 12
  How much do you drink? 14
  Which has the most? 15
  Associations 16
  Is it a problem? 17

Hidden food allergy
  Are you allergic? 19
  What do you eat? 20
  What suits me? 21

Recipes 23

From mood to food 24

Food problems? Some solutions 25

Food tasting 26

Taking supplements 28

The Food & Mood Project library 29

Some useful contacts 31

Feedback! 32

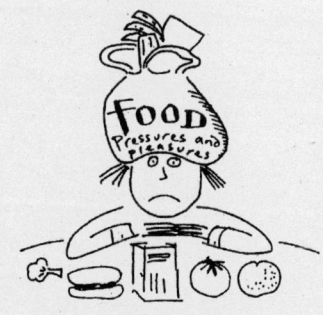

Foreword

Since 1997 the Mind Millennium Awards have enabled over 500 Award winners and some 200 projects to both raise the issues surrounding mental health and to benefit their communities.

Amanda Geary is one such Award winner and her workbook has some very positive information and advice for all of us around diet, nutrition and mental health. This publication will go a long way to combat the ignorance surrounding the positive effects nutritional therapy can bring to people.

The whole project turned out to be both exciting and innovative, attracting much interest from the national media. The book will add to the ever growing body of evidence that supports the importance of diet and nutrition in mental health.

Ray Davies
Mind Millennium Awards Team, Mind, London

Acknowledgements

The Millennium Commission and the mental health charity Mind for the Mind Millennium Award that made the Project possible.

Andy Porter, Director, Brighton & Hove Mind, and Helen Bashford and Terry Bell-Halliwell at Threshold Women's Counselling, Brighton, for their support of the Project, particularly in its early days.

Les Moore and Fiona Saunders at Natural Health Foods/Wholefood Express in Brighton for providing a home for the Project.

Joy Dillon and Kate Benson at East Sussex, Brighton & Hove Health Promotion for their continued interest and support.

Most importantly, the 54 women who took part in the Project by attending the workshops and sharing their experiences. The Project depended wholly on your contributions for its success. Thank you.

Apologies to the many others wanting a place in the workshops but who had to be turned away due to lack of space. I hope you will be able to gain some benefit through using this Workbook.

Welcome to the Food & Mood Workbook

This Workbook is intended to provide a starting point for individuals or groups who wish to explore their relationship with food. I have no doubt that what we eat and drink has an important part to play in how we feel – mentally and emotionally as well as physically. In this Workbook you will find some signposts to guide your journey and hopefully discover just how intimate is our connection with food.

The Mind Millenium Award funded Food & Mood workshops contained much information and advice, only some of which can be reproduced here. In addition to the information about foods you will also find examples of the thought-provoking exercises which aimed to increase awareness of the feelings associated with eating and drinking.

The Project's success depended entirely on the 50 or so women who were able to take part by attending the workshops and sharing their experiences and I would like to express my gratitude for their committed and enthusiastic participation. These women have much food-related wisdom to share and this Workbook also contains some of their written contributions.

Finally, although the Food & Mood Project was originally set up as a service for women, the recommendations in this Workbook also apply to men and to children.

Amanda Geary
The Food & Mood Project

> *Let food be your medicine and medicine be your food.*
> HIPPOCRATES

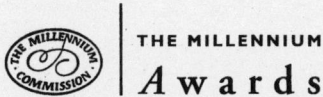

THE MILLENNIUM Awards

The Food and Mood Workbook has been produced by The Food & Mood Project, an 18-month community initiative funded from an award made by the Millennium Commission working in conjunction with Mind, the mental health charity. Mind Millennium Awards are recognised as an 'accolade rewarding imagination, aspiration, achievement' and were granted to enable activities that would not have otherwise been possible, which demonstrated a benefit to the community and which raised the profile of mental health.

Food & mood and you

When it comes to your relationship with food, how well do you know yourself? Here are some of the questions we consider in Food & Mood workshops.

1 What is your favourite food?
2 What is your favourite meal?
3 What foods do you dislike?
4 On a usual day what are you likely to eat?
5 Complete the sentence:

When I feel _____ I like to eat/drink _____

6 Complete the sentence:

When I eat/drink _____ I feel _____

7 What habits, routines and rituals do you have around food?

8 Think of a word or phrase that describes what food means (or meant) to you
   a) as a child:
   b) as an adult:
   c) as a food provider or parent:

9 In your experience, how is food used?
   - to show love
   - to show disapproval
   - as a bribe
   - to relieve boredom
   - as a comfort
   - as a reward/incentive
   - instead of giving attention
   - to upset someone?

10 How do *you* use food?

Notice how your answers change with time.

Acknowledgement: questions 8 and 9 are reproduced from *Women, Food and Health* produced by Mancunian Community Nutrition.

> I found the session on blood sugar levels and sugars in foods has really shed light on a murky area where, since childhood, I have struggled to be at peace with myself and what I eat.
>
> *Food & Mood Project participant*

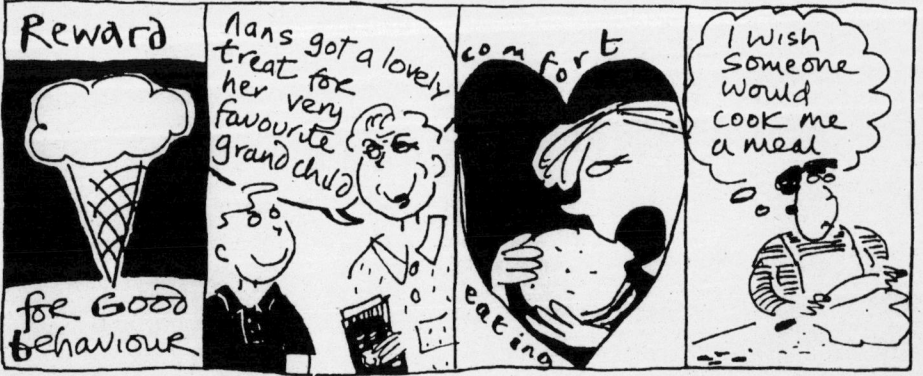

Changing what you eat

This Food & Mood Workbook invites you to consider the possibility of a link between what you eat and how you feel – mentally and emotionally – and then provides you with suggestions for some changes you could make (based on what other people have found useful) in order to explore that relationship.

Finding the diet that's right for you is the aim and it is important to remember that we all have different needs and what suits one person may not be appropriate for another. Therefore the process of discovery encourages individuals to take control of the exploration yet at the same time be prepared to learn from others' experiences.

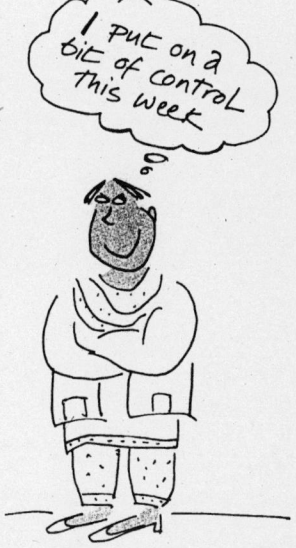

"As long as you derive inner help and comfort from anything, you should keep it. If you were to give it up in a mood of self-sacrifice or out of a stern sense of duty, you would continue to want it back, and that unsatisfied want would make trouble for you. Only give up a thing when you want some other condition so much that the thing no longer has any attraction for you."
Ghandi (quoted in *Voluntary Simplicity* by Duane Elgin)

Changing what you eat invariably involves eating or drinking less of some things and more of others. It is preferable – and easier – to cut out something if you can anticipate a benefit from doing so and also if you are able to replace it with something else. It is also very helpful if you can enlist the support of family, friends or colleagues at work.

Before we can make changes to our diet to improve our health we need to be aware of what we are already eating and drinking and how we are feeling. The effect of making changes can be quite dramatic. Sometimes the benefits are less obvious and it is only when we look back on how things used to be, that we can appreciate what's been achieved. One useful way to start the process of exploration is to keep a food & mood diary.

I used to be addicted to chocolate ...

I have given up before. Chocolate is not seen as a 'serious' addiction. It helped a lot to be in the Food & Mood group and receive the support from the other women. Amanda suggests that you replace whatever you're giving up with something else, and I think I've replaced chocolate with looking more at the world and noticing things.

So there is life after chocolate.

*Dorothy Stuart
Food & Mood Project participant*

Keeping a food & mood diary

This needs to be kept for at least a week and ideally one month. The reasons for keeping a food & mood diary are:

- **To find out exactly what you are eating and drinking – which may not be quite what you think!**
- **To identify anything in your diet that could be affecting your moods.**

Aim to record what you eat and drink as it happens rather than trying to remember afterwards – it is easier to carry your food & mood diary with you. At first the idea of writing down everything that passes your lips may seem a chore but, hopefully, after a while you will be able to enjoy the process of reflecting upon what you are doing and how you are feeling and see it as an opportunity to become more self aware.

The food & mood diary works best if it is kept in a clear and methodical manner and a suggestion for its layout together with an example of what it may look like is given below.

The more information the diary contains the more useful it is likely to be. It can be helpful to score physical and emotional symptoms, perhaps by rating them on a 1-10 scale where 10 is the worst possible and 1 is very mild.

When you look back over the diary you may notice, for example, that you felt worse whenever you skipped breakfast or that you felt less irritable after you had a coffee. This greater awareness of the possible relationship between your food and your moods is the first important step to making appropriate changes.

Food & Mood Diary

Time & date	What I eat/drink	How I feel physically	How I feel emotionally
Mon 12			
8am	coffee (black, 2 sugars)	tired/aching (8)	irritable (6)
10am	2 doughnuts	ditto	irritable (3)
11am	coffee (black, 2 sugars)	OK	anxious (5)

The stressors of life

Our ability to cope with stress determines how healthy we are. Put another way, our health can be seen as a measure of how well we adapt to the various stressors which are all around us.

Stressors are, quite literally, things that can put a stress on a person and if we exceed our capacity to cope with them we begin to fall ill.

All of us live intimately with our environment and our relationship with our surroundings needs to be harmonious if we are to remain healthy. It can often help to take a more holistic view of health and consider the whole picture as well as looking at individual pieces of the jigsaw whilst we search for a solution to the problems of ill health. The whole picture, when considering our ability to cope with stress and the things that cause us stress, is known as the 'total load'.

We can think of our ability to adapt to these stressors as being like a bath, with each of us represented by a different sized bath according to our inherited and acquired characteristics.

Food related stressors include:
caffeine
chocolate
refined sugars
food allergens
food additives
some natural chemicals in food
fertilisers
pesticides
herbicides
antibiotics
growth promoters
pollutants (such as xenoestrogens, PCBs, dioxins)
micro-organisms
parasites
natural toxicants (eg mycotoxins)
and, probably, GMOs

Mood related symptoms include:
anxiety, depression, mood swings, cravings, PMS

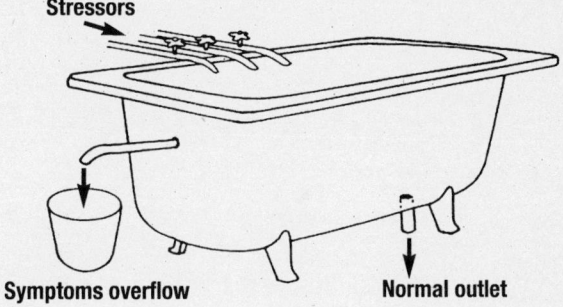

Stressors

Symptoms overflow   **Normal outlet**

Into the bath is flowing all the various influences upon our spiritual, mental, emotional and physical health. The bath has an outlet (unplugged) and the capacity to cope with a certain amount without any difficulty. But if the total flow going into the bath – the total load – is more than the bath can contain, then the bath will start to overflow. Symptoms of disease, be they physical or mental, emotional or spiritual, are a sign that the person has exceeded their ability to deal with the total load of stressors in their environment. The greater the overflow from the bath, the worse are the symptoms.

This Food & Mood Workbook describes just three possible food stressors which are found in most people's daily diets. As far as explaining mental health is concerned, they cannot be the whole picture but they are important pieces of the jigsaw and certainly play a part in contributing to the total load flowing into the bath.

Acknowledgement: The 'bath' is reproduced with permission and is taken from *Allergy: a practical guide to coping* by J Maberly & H Anthony, 1989, The Crowood Press, UK.

Recipe

Easy risotto with onion and bean salad

Ingredients
50g brown rice (per person)
185g can tuna in brine
400g can peeled plum tomatoes
300g can chickpeas
326g can sweetcorn

Method
Put rice in a pan of boiling, salted water, stir gently and reduce heat. Cover and simmer for 15-20 mins until tender. Rinse and drain well.

While the rice is cooking, drain all other ingredients including tomatoes. Mix rice, tuna, tomatoes, chickpeas and sweetcorn together. Season with one of the following: garlic, soy sauce, chilli sauce, Worcester sauce, or any other of your choice.

Serving suggestion
Serve hot or cold with a green salad.
Alternatively, peel and slice and blanche a large onion. Mix it with a 300g can of either cannellini or borlotti beans and serve as an accompaniment.

Marian Saunders
Food & Mood Project participant

Food & mood – a personal view

My main goal during the course was to begin to take active steps to reduce migraine and headaches and the actions I have taken were prompted by the course and so far these seem to have helped. I cut down on stimulants, especially tea, coffee and chocolate. I began to take supplements which included a multi mineral and vitamin, B-complex, sage leaf, St John's wort, starflower and vitamin C. I also began to keep a diary of everything – yes everything – that I ate each day. This was quite revealing. I kept this up for a total of six weeks and this proved to be a straightforward system for monitoring eating habits. The most useful and at times alarming part was putting a highlighter pen through the items that I needed to avoid or cut down on and the more marker pen I used ... A real benefit of the course was being in a group, sitting together sharing ideas, talking about food and health-related experiences and most of all: sharing food.

Deborah Morley
Food & Mood Project participant

Quiz: Am I sugar sensitive?

How many of the following can you relate to? Tick the boxes that apply.

- ☐ I often feel dizzy, shaky, faint, fuzzy headed or have difficulty concentrating
- ☐ I usually feel drowsy or tired during the day
- ☐ I get headaches quite often
- ☐ I sweat a lot during the night or day
- ☐ I am often anxious, fearful or depressed
- ☐ I get moody or irritable, angry or feel aggressive unexpectedly
- ☐ I get stressed out easily
- ☐ I tend to put on weight easily
- ☐ I tend to graze on food throughout the day
- ☐ I often feel I need a tea, coffee, cola, cigarette or alcoholic drink
- ☐ I've got a sweet tooth – I like eating sweet things
- ☐ I really like eating bread, cereal, pasta

A day in the life of ... you

Draw a line on the following chart that shows the highs and lows of your moods and energy levels during a typical day. You could also mark on the chart when you eat, drink, smoke or take medications.

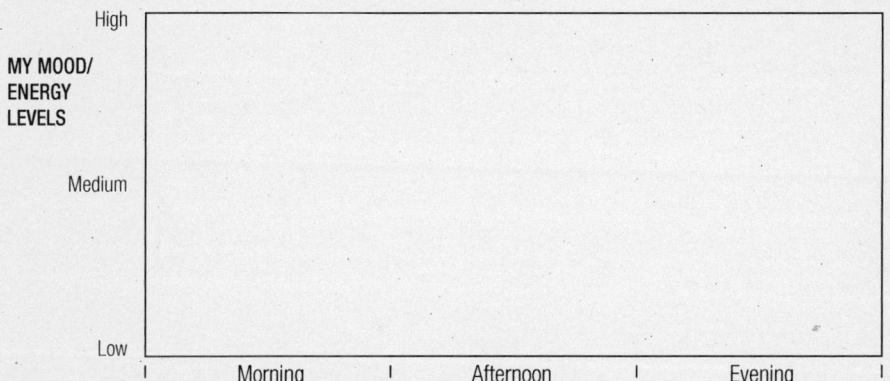

Now turn the page to find out what your answers to the quiz mean and also to interpret your mood/energy levels chart.

Is sugar sensitivity a problem?

Sugar sensitivity quiz: the statements listed in the quiz are symptoms of sugar sensitivity and the more you ticked the more likely you are to be sugar sensitive. The brain is the organ most sensitive to a change in blood sugar level – too little glucose produces fatigue, confusion, irritability and aggression while too much may result in loss of consciousness.

Mood and energy levels chart: compare your chart from the previous page with the following which equates fluctuations in energy levels and moods with fluctuations in blood sugar levels.

Blood sugar levels of someone who is sugar sensitive

The bodies of sugar sensitive people have a stronger reaction to eating sugary foods. For these people, increases in blood sugar that occur after eating tend to be higher and more rapid than for non-sugar sensitive people. The healthy pancreas releases insulin to get the excess sugar out of the blood, and the sugar high is followed by a steep drop in blood sugar level. Blood sugar levels are then too low and a hit of sugar is needed quickly. Unfortunately for the sugar sensitive person who eats fast energy releasing foods the blood sugar levels go shooting up again. This roller-coaster ride in blood sugar levels often results in similar highs and lows of mood and energy.

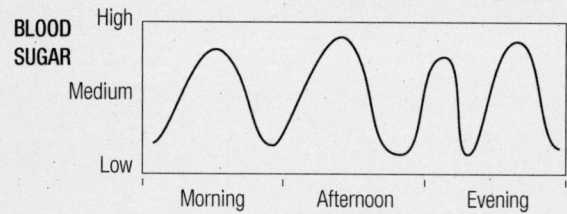

Someone with low sugar sensitivity or on a sugar-free diet

The blood sugar curve of a person who is not sugar sensitive, or of a sugar sensitive person who eats only slow energy releasing foods, has no extreme peaks or troughs. It rises gently in response to eating something and falls slowly as the sugar is used for energy. Blood sugar levels are fairly stable and predictable.

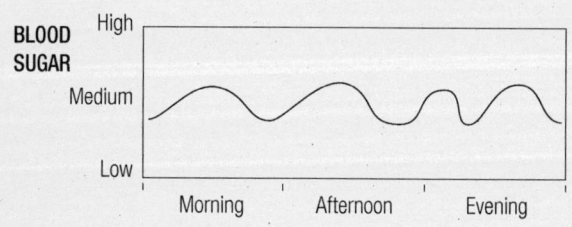

Further reading: *Potatoes not Prozac* by Kathleen DesMaisons PhD, 1998, Simon & Schuster UK Ltd.

Sugar

How to manage sugar sensitivity

If you think you might be sugar sensitive and would like to iron out the highs and lows of energy and mood and experience life on a more even keel there are a number of changes that you can make to achieve this which can be effective within weeks or even days.

The most important change is to eat foods that don't contain concentrated sugars and which release their energy slowly over a longer period of time. Sugary foods tend to send your blood sugar level up very quickly and are best avoided. Instead, slow-releasing foods keep you going for longer and help you to avoid the peaks and troughs of fluctuating blood sugar levels which can create a rollercoaster ride of emotions.

Choosing slow-releasing foods

1 Replace 'white' foods with 'brown'

FROM WHITE
eg:
white rice
white bread
white pasta
french baguette bread
bagel

TO BROWN
eg:
brown rice
wholemeal bread
wholemeal pasta
pastries/cakes with wholemeal flour
oatcake biscuits

Like the tortoise, slow and steady does it better when it comes to energy-releasing foods

2 Choose foods with a low Glycaemic Index

The GI of a food shows the effect of that food on blood sugar, compared to pure glucose which is given a score of 100. Foods with a lower GI score do not raise blood sugar levels as much as foods with a higher score and are therefore preferable. Some low GI foods to choose are given below.

FOOD	GI SCORE
	0-60=low 60-100=high
Digestive biscuits (plain)	59
Basmati rice	58
Pitta bread	57
Meusli	56
Sweetcorn/Popcorn	55
Sweet potato	54
Baked beans	48
Porridge oats	42
Wholegrain rye bread (eg Pumpernickel)	41
Apple/Pear	38
Spaghetti (wholemeal)	37
Apricots (dried)	31

Further reading: *The GI Factor* by Dr A Leeds et al, 1996. Hodder & Stoughton.

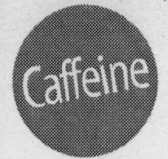

Quiz

Decide whether the following are true or false   TRUE   FALSE

1. Caffeine is found in chocolate, tea, coffee, and cola. ☐ ☐

2. Caffeine is the most widely consumed stimulant drug in the world. ☐ ☐

3. Caffeine can be bought in pills from the chemists. ☐ ☐

4. Caffeine consumption is followed by an increase in blood pressure and adrenalin production and can encourage glucose intolerance through its simulatory effect on the adrenal glands. ☐ ☐

5. Caffeine is absorbed quickly and stays in your body for about 1 hour. ☐ ☐

6. If you're on the Pill caffeine lasts longer in your body. ☐ ☐

7. Drinking coffee can contribute to osteoporosis. ☐ ☐

8. Caffeine is a diuretic (urine producing) so if you drink too much you can become dehydrated. ☐ ☐

9. Caffeine can make you constipated. ☐ ☐

10. Caffeine can help with a hangover. ☐ ☐

11. Drinking tea could make you anaemic. ☐ ☐

12. Caffeine taken on a regular basis can lead to addiction which means you need to take more to get the same effect. ☐ ☐

13. 'Decaff' drinks means all the caffeine has been taken out. ☐ ☐

14. 'Decaff' coffee can be made using dry cleaning chemicals. ☐ ☐

	TRUE	FALSE

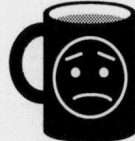

15 Too much caffeine can cause anxiety, nervousness and depression. ☐ ☐

16 Not enough caffeine can make you irritable and cause difficulty concentrating. ☐ ☐

17 PMS can be helped by a caffeine-free diet. ☐ ☐

18 Coming off of caffeine 'cold turkey' takes 3 weeks. ☐ ☐

19 You can treat caffeine withdrawal symptoms such as a headache by using the 'hair of the dog' approach, taking sips of coffee or tea. ☐ ☐

20 Coffee enemas are sometimes used for treating cancer. ☐ ☐

Answers

1 True.
2 True.
3 True: Caffeine is found in painkillers and flu remedies.
4 True.
5 False: Caffeine is absorbed quickly and reaches peak levels in about an hour but can remain in the body for 2-12 hours.
6 True.
7 True: Excessive caffeine consumption depletes the body's stores of calcium.
8 True.
9 True & False: Coffee has a mild laxative effect but because of caffeine's diuretic effect it can contribute to constipation.
10 True & False: Coffee may in fact aggravate a hangover by increasing dehydration due to its diuretic effect.
11 True: The consumption of tea or coffee within one hour of a meal can reduce iron absorption by up to 80%.
12 True.
13 False: By law instant 'decaff' coffee must have no more than 0.3% caffeine which means there can still be some caffeine in 'decaff'.
14 True: Decaffeination can use an organic solvent such as methylene chloride or ethyl acetate which are also used in paint strippers, aerosols and dry cleaning solutions so there is concern about the possibility of these solvent residues remaining in the end product. Alternative methods use carbon dioxide or water.
15 True: These are symptoms of 'caffeinism'.
16 True: These are some symptoms of withdrawal from caffeine.
17 True: Also, low fertility – 5 mugs of coffee per day has been shown to produce a 60% reduction in fertility.
18 False: The worst of the withdrawal symptoms are usually over after 3-5 days.
19 True: Better still, drink plenty of water to help the detoxification process.
20 True: Pioneered by the late Dr Gerson in the 1950's.

Further reading: *Secret Ingredients*, P Cox & P Brusseau, 1997, Bantam Books.

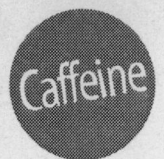

Caffeine

How much do you drink?

Complete the following table then compare your daily intake with the women who took part in the Food & Mood Project

Number of portions per day

Tea (including decaff) ☐ cups

Coffee (including decaff) ☐ cups

Chocolate (bars and drink) ☐ small bars/cups

Cola (plus similar drinks) ☐ glasses/cans

The table below gives the percentage of women in the Food & Mood Project who drank cups of tea, coffee, cola (or other caffeine-containing fizzy drinks) or ate chocolate, and the amount they consumed, measured as the number of portions per day.

Number of portions consumed per day

	0 ZERO	1-3 LOW	3-6 MEDIUM	6+ HIGH
Tea (including decaff)	34%	47%	11%	8%
Coffee (including decaff)	29%	55%	11%	5%
Chocolate (bars and drink)	45%	50%	5%	0%
Cola (plus similar drinks)	55%	40%	5%	0%

- Taken as a group, most of the women in the Food & Mood Project drank 1-3 cups of tea and between 1 and 3 cups of coffee per day (individual women may have drunk either tea or coffee and not both).

- Half of the women in the Food & Mood Project ate at least one bar of chocolate or drank one cup of hot chocolate every day.

- Most of the women who took part in the project did not drink, on a regular basis, any cola or fizzy drinks containing caffeine.

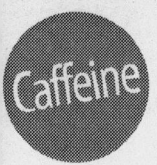

Caffeine

Which has the most?

Rank these 12 drinks in descending order of caffeine content, starting with the drink that contains the most caffeine:

____ a cup of instant coffee

____ a fizzy drink containing the herb guarana

____ a cup of tea made with a teabag

____ a can of cola

____ a cup of filter coffee

____ a bar of plain chocolate

____ a cup of 'hot chocolate'

____ a bar of milk chocolate

____ a cup of tea made with loose leaf tea

____ a cup of 'green' tea

____ a cup of 'decaff'

____ a cup of 'Red Bush' herbal tea

Recognise addiction

Satisfying cravings of any kind (nicotine, chocolate, caffeine, alcohol) is no way to help yourself feel calm. Recognise addictions for what they are, and find an alternative. Then you can be calm.

From *The Little Book of Calm*, – contributed by Sonia Peterson, Food & Mood Project participant

Answers

1. a cup of filter coffee contains the most caffeine (the average mug contains around 100mg)
2. instant coffee
3. loose leaf tea
4. tea made with a bag (tea averages around 40mg caffeine per cup)
5. green tea (a beneficial antioxidant containing polyphenols – potent free radical scavengers with some anti-carginogenic action)
6. cola (the average can contains around 23mg caffeine while some energy drinks have four times the amount)
7. plain chocolate
8. milk chocolate (plain chocolate has 40mg caffeine per 100g – nearly three times as much as milk chocolate)
9. a cup of 'hot chocolate'
10. a cup of 'decaff'
11. a fizzy drink containing the herb guarana (a South American herb closely related to caffeine but possibly not as toxic)
12. a cup of Red Bush herbal tea (this is naturally caffeine free although it does contain tannin, an 'antinutrient' which binds to minerals, such as iron and zinc, in the gut thus preventing their absorption)

Main references:
Which? Way to Heath Oct 1995 and *Health Which?* Feb 1999

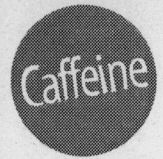

Caffeine

These are the things the Food & Mood Project participants might think of if you mention to them the words 'coffee',' tea' or 'chocolate'.

What do you think of?

Associations

old ladies · chat · wake up · Brief Encounter · fixes me · grown up · conversation · instant · routine · take a break · sober up · guilt · friends · insomnia · crisis · after dinner · bingeing · addiction · poison · fattening · smell · buzz · in front of the telly · cigarettes · social · headache · mood swings · ritual · liquid cake · aroma · lift · comfort · temptation · relaxation · my favourite mug · habit · prize · indulgence · elevenses · in my mouth · hangover · trendy · sophisticated · irresistible · solves the problem · cosmopolitan · stimulant · thirsty · feel nice · stress cure? · pick-me-up · cosy · bonding · when something goes wrong · fitting in · continental · pleasant · staying power · nurturing · sex · breakfast · texture

---

Food & Mood feedback

I've been able to use the workshops to focus on what my food intake involves and to explore possible changes and beneficial ways of eating. Its been quite an illuminating experience and has presented me with a lot of information. I've found the pace and emphasis of the whole group to be respectful and non-invasive. Absolutely non-scary!

Claire – Food & Mood Project participant

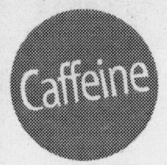

Is it a problem?

There may be something about your health that you'd like to change – perhaps anxiety, depression, mood swings, cravings, PMS – which could be achieved by cutting down or coming off caffeine. Yet there are advantages as well as disadvantages to consuming the caffeine found in coffee, tea, chocolate and cola drinks.

What are the important considerations for you? (If you're stuck have a look at the *Caffeine quiz* on page 12 and *Caffeine associations* on page 16). You could then write your ideas in the diagram below.

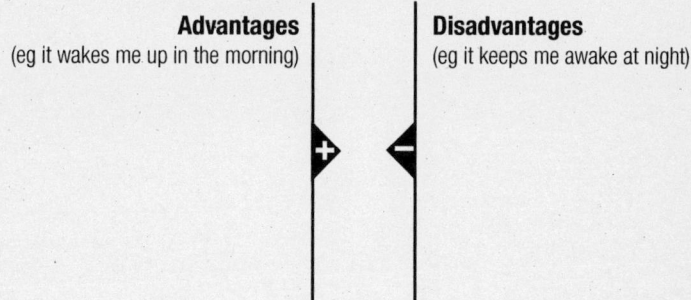

CONSUMING CAFFEINE?

Advantages (eg it wakes me up in the morning)

Disadvantages (eg it keeps me awake at night)

After weighing up the pros and cons of consuming caffeine you may conclude that you need more information.

The only way to be certain of the effect that caffeine is having on you is to cut it down or cut it out – and find out for yourself.

You will then be in a better position to decide if, when and how you want to use this potent drug, based on your own experience.

Coming off caffeine

If you do decide to cut down or cut out caffeine, here are some hints to help you:

- Start by listing the sources of caffeine in your diet and how much you are consuming (see pages 14 and 15).

- Decide if you want to stop suddenly or wean yourself off gradually (if you stop suddenly you are likely to experience withdrawal symptoms for 3-5 days; if you wean yourself off gradually any withdrawal symptoms will be lessened).

- Stock up on alternative drinks (see *Food tasting* on page 26) and have a go!

YOU ARE WHAT YOU EAT

Nutrition – a personal view

Nutrition is the foundation of life – ask anyone who has been without food. When we have nourishment we have the ability to feel with our whole being and to see the beauty of life. We all know the saying 'you are what you eat' but do we really understand how to nourish ourselves?

It is our responsibility to educate ourselves so that we can nourish our bodies for optimum health. But not just the physical body. The heart, mind, soul and spirit also need food and with this comes true freedom because we become less cloudy and begin to know the meaning of life.

We need to recognise that nourishment is something that doesn't just exist on the physical plane – the fact that so many people eat 3-4 meals a day but still feel empty and dissatisfied confirms this. We need to relax in order to be active, we have to calmly sit and eat and chew our food to liquid, we have to breath deeply into our bellies and we have to meditate, take time out to stop and clear our thoughts, then we will have renewed strength. We have to have positive thoughts and do our work with happiness or change our jobs! All these things help us to assimilate our food properly.

When we are nourished on all levels we don't have to suffer ill health or stress related problems, we will be able to give and receive love and have joy in our lives and our world. The universe is one symphony and we are all part of the orchestra.

Pure food helps your body not get in the way of spiritual growth. Our body is a temple that houses a beautiful light. If we keep the windows clean, it can shine out.

Light & gratitude.

Amanda Wright
Food & Mood Project participant

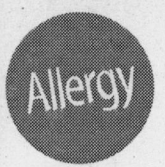

You will probably already know if you have any 'classic' allergies to foods because the effect on your body of eating these foods will be very quick and probably quite dramatic. However, it is possible that you may have hidden food allergies or other food sensitivities which are less obvious in the effects they produce but which, nonetheless, can be having an extremely disabling influence upon your health.

Are you allergic?

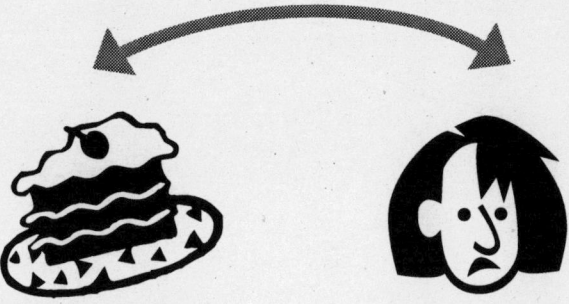

FROM FOOD
In neuro-psychological illnesses, the foods most commonly found linked with symptoms are:

wheat
milk & milk products
yeast
sugar
coffee
chocolate
oranges
egg
tomato
corn
soya
additives

TO MOOD
Neuro-psychological symptoms or illnesses which can be made worse or which can be caused by foods include:

depression
mood changes
behavioural disorders
anxiety & panic attacks
hyperactivity
poor memory, concentration
sleep disorders
migraine
poor co-ordination
numbness, tingling, restless legs
fatigue
seasonal affective disorder
eating disorders

What is food to one man may be fierce poison to another LUCRETIUS

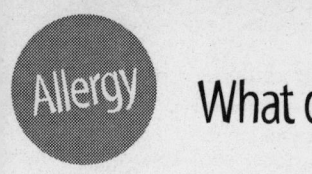

What do you eat?

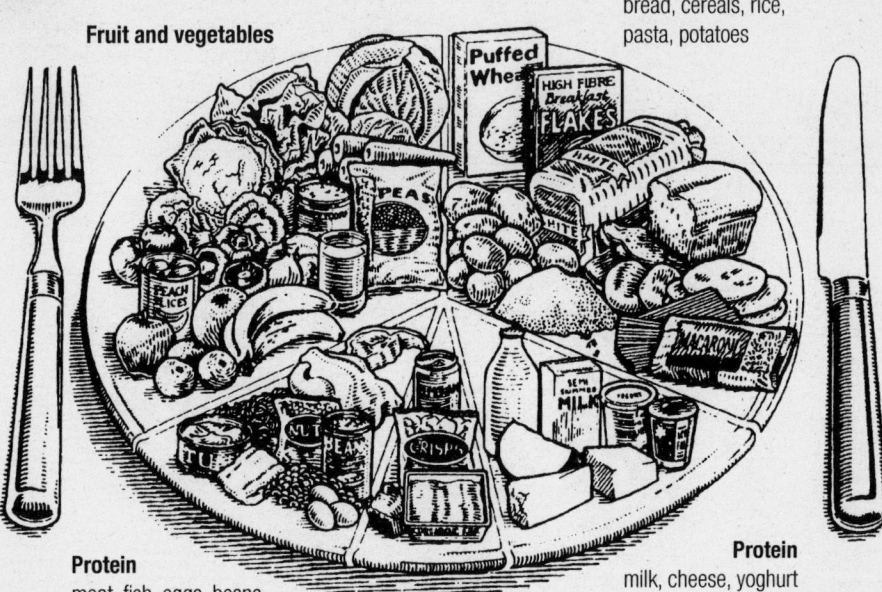

Fruit and vegetables

Carbohydrates
bread, cereals, rice,
pasta, potatoes

Protein
meat, fish, eggs, beans

Fatty and sugary food

Protein
milk, cheese, yoghurt

The plate above is divided up to show the main types of foods and the different proportions which are recommended by the UK Health Education Authority as being suitable for most adults and children over the age of two years.

The largest two segments are carbohydrate-based foods (bread, cereals, rice, pasta, potatoes) and fruit and vegetables. The foods providing protein are divided into two segments: meat, fish, eggs and beans, and milk, cheese and yoghurt. The smallest segment is for the foods that contain fat (such as in butter and crisps) and sugars (such as fizzy drinks and cakes).

However, each of us has unique biochemical and nutritional needs. These needs vary at different times in our lives and the diet that keeps one person healthy can make another person ill. It is therefore important to find out what suits us now – as individuals.

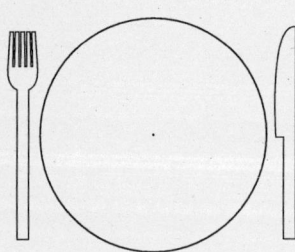

If you grouped together the main categories of food and drink that you usually consume and represented them as segments of a 'plate', what would the overall balance of your diet look like?

Acknowledgement: food plate illustration reproduced with permission from Sustain: the alliance for better food & farming.

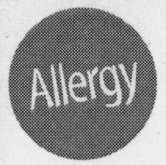

What suits me?

The suspects
If you would like to find out if you are sensitive to any of the foods you are eating you need to draw up a list of suspects. You may already have some suspicions as to the foods that may be 'disagreeing' with you in some way, and these could be your prime suspects. Also worth further investigation are anything you eat on a daily basis or several times a week. As you draw up your list, make sure you include the foods that you really enjoy eating (which you may even crave on occasions) and be aware that the initial enjoyment these foods can provide may be distracting you from their unpleasant effects which can be experienced up to several days later. Another rich source of clues can be found in the experiences of other people – the foods most often associated with psychological symptoms are listed on page 19.

The investigation
Whilst it is tempting to investigate all the suspects together, many people find that changing much of their diet all at once is counterproductive as the stress of doing so adds – rather than reduces – their 'total load' (see page 7). Also, changing your diet can produce withdrawal symptoms which are easier to manage if you decide to 'chip away', one by one, at the changes you want to make.

There are three ways you can conduct your investigation of suspect foods:

1. **Reduce** the amount of a suspect food you eat, replacing it with something nutritionally similar.

2. Increase the variety of foods you eat and '**rotate**' the alternatives'. The alternatives can include the suspect food(s) so long as they are each eaten only once every few days – perhaps just on one day in every 4-5 days or, if its easier to plan, just on one day a week.

3. Use the process of '**elimination and challenge**'. Put simply, the elimination and challenge method involves cutting out a suspect food (and replacing it with something nutritionally similar) for approximately 14 days – the elimination stage – and then reintroducing it in the challenge stage. This process needs care, particularly when the body is 'challenged' with the eliminated food. At the challenge stage, any sensitivity you may have to the suspect food under investigation can be increased, so that when you introduce the food, symptoms are produced which – for some people – can be difficult to deal with. Alternatively symptoms can become delayed and then easily missed or not associated with the food eaten.

Whichever method you choose it is made a lot easier if you can enlist the support of family, friends, colleagues and, ideally, a health care professional experienced in using these methods. Keeping a food & mood diary of what you eat when, and also how you feel, provides a vital source of useful information which can otherwise be forgotten or dismissed as being insignificant.

CONTINUED ON NEXT PAGE...

Further reading: please refer to the 'Allergy' section of the Food & Mood Library on page 29.

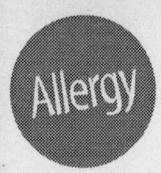

Allergy

Dealing with the culprits

Once you are reasonably confident that any improvements in your symptoms are related to the alterations in your diet, you will need to decide whether the benefits you experience are worth the effort of sustaining these changes in the long term. If you *are* able to keep going with your new diet, you may well find that your sensitivities lessen over time as your body enjoys the 'holiday' from the foods it didn't like and starts to heal itself.

Changing what you eat, whether for a short time to identify problem foods or as a longer term strategy for healing, involves a certain amount of planning and reorganisation of routines. You may find that you need to find new places to shop and buy the alternatives you are substituting. One benefit of this process is that you will discover a greater variety of new foods to enjoy that you may not have otherwise tried.

The more you are able to reduce the amount of offending foods in your diet, the more benefits you will experience. To manage this you will need to become a 'food detective' and learn to decipher food labels. In the box on the right are some clues to help you with the most common offenders: wheat and milk/products.

Substitutes and alternatives

Nutritionally similar substitutes for bread and other foods containing wheat include breads and recipes that use rye flour, corn/maize or rice flour instead. Alternatives to cows milk include 'Rice Dream' (made from rice), soya 'milk', oat 'milk', almond 'milk'. These 'milks' are not suitable as cows milk substitutes for babies and very young children. *Food tasting* on pages 26-27 also provides some suggestions for alternative foods to try.

Wheat

If you are testing for a wheat sensitivity by cutting down, rotating or eliminating wheat from your diet, this will include most types of bread and all foods containing wheat. Hidden sources of wheat (and you may discover others) are described as 'flour', 'starch', 'gluten', 'rusk', 'cereal filler/protein', 'plant/vegetable protein/gum', 'wheatgerm', 'wheatberries', 'bran'.

Note also that bulgar wheat, semolina and couscous are all derived from wheat but that, despite the name, buckwheat is not related to wheat and therefore can be eaten.

Milk

If you are testing for a milk sensitivity by cutting down, rotating or eliminating milk from your diet, you will need to check foods for milk hidden as 'whey', 'curd', 'lactose', 'casein', 'lactalbumin', 'lactoglobulin', 'milk solids', 'milk fats'.

Note also that the following do not contain milk and need not be avoided in a milk-free diet: 'lactic acid', 'lactate', 'lactylate'.

Further reading: Brostoff, J & Gamlin, L (1989) *The Complete Guide to Food Allergy and Intolerance* Bloomsbury, London and other books listed in the allergy section of the Food & Mood Library on page 29.

Recipes

Millet burgers

3 oz dry millet
1 med onion – finely chopped
3 oz cheese – grated
1 tblspn chopped parsley
2oz bread crumbs
1/2 tspn thyme
good pinch mustard powder
pepper & salt
1 egg – separated
2 tblspn plain wholemeal flour
oil for frying

Method
To cook the millet: heat a teaspoon of oil in a saucepan and lightly toast the millet in it. Pour on 1/2 pint water, bring to the boil, stir once and cover the pan. Cook for approx 20 mins until the water is absorbed and the millet grains are fluffy. Cool on a large plate. In a bowl, combine the onion, grated cheese, cooked millet, herbs, seasoning and egg yolk. Beat egg white lightly and set aside. Shape mixture into six burgers. Dip in flour, then egg white and roll in the bread crumbs. Shallow fry until brown on both sides or grill on a piece of foil for about 10-15 mins.

Food & Mood Project participant

Oat rissoles

Eat hot with vegetable, cold with salad. Ideal for freezing.

2lbs oats
2 onions, grated
7-8 cloves garlic
mixed herbs
1-2 eggs
3-4 tblspns soya flour
grated raw carrot (if desired)

Method
Mix all ingredients thoroughly. Add marmite to make a flexible mixture. Place in tins (fairy cake individual tins) and /or pyrex dishes. Bake in oven until brown for approx 1 1/2 hours.

Irene Gould – Food & Mood Project participant

From mood to food

The relationship between food and mood works both ways and there are very many factors influencing what we eat and drink. It is helpful to be aware of as many of these as possible so that we can take greater control of them and start to make more informed choices about our diet.

What influences what we eat and drink?
This question was considered by the Food & Mood Project along with our ideas for making changes for the better. We found that most of us had some idea as to how we could improve our diets but that we also experienced many blocks that appeared to be preventing us from actually making those changes.

Blocks to better eating

How many of these can you identify with?

A SWEET TOOTH	IT WAS IN THE FRIDGE	NOTHING IN THE FRIDGE	PERSISTENT THOUGHTS
SOCIAL OCCASIONS	NEEDING A TREAT	ADS ON TV	ALCOHOL LOWERING INHIBITIONS
OTHER PEOPLE	COOKING FOR OTHERS	COOKING FOR ONE	WANTING TO PLEASE	HABIT
LONELINESS	BOREDOM	DISTRACTION	NOT WANTING TO WASTE FOOD	FEELING DEPRIVED
EATING WHEN OUT OR TRAVELLING	DEPRESSION	TOO BUSY	CRAVINGS	THE TASTE
TEMPTATION WHEN SHOPPING	STRESSED	IN A HURRY	NOT WANTING TO 'MAKE A FUSS'
LACK OF £££	DON'T WANT TO BE 'DIFFERENT'	NEEDING COMFORT	THE SMELL	FATIGUE
WANTING TO PLEASE	DON'T WANT TO BE LEFT OUT	PREMENSTRUAL	LACK OF WILL POWER
REBELLION	HUNGER – NEED A QUICK FIX	PLEASURE	DESIRE	NEED TO CONCENTRATE
CONFUSION ABOUT WHAT'S RIGHT	ORAL GRATIFICATION	PROCRASTINATION	FEELING ILL
CAN'T GET WHAT'S RIGHT	CAN'T BE BOTHERED	INDIVIDUAL TV DINNERS	FAMILY PRESSURE
HAVING TO PROVE I HAVEN'T GOT A PROBLEM WITH FOOD	LACK OF PLANNING	NO CHOICE

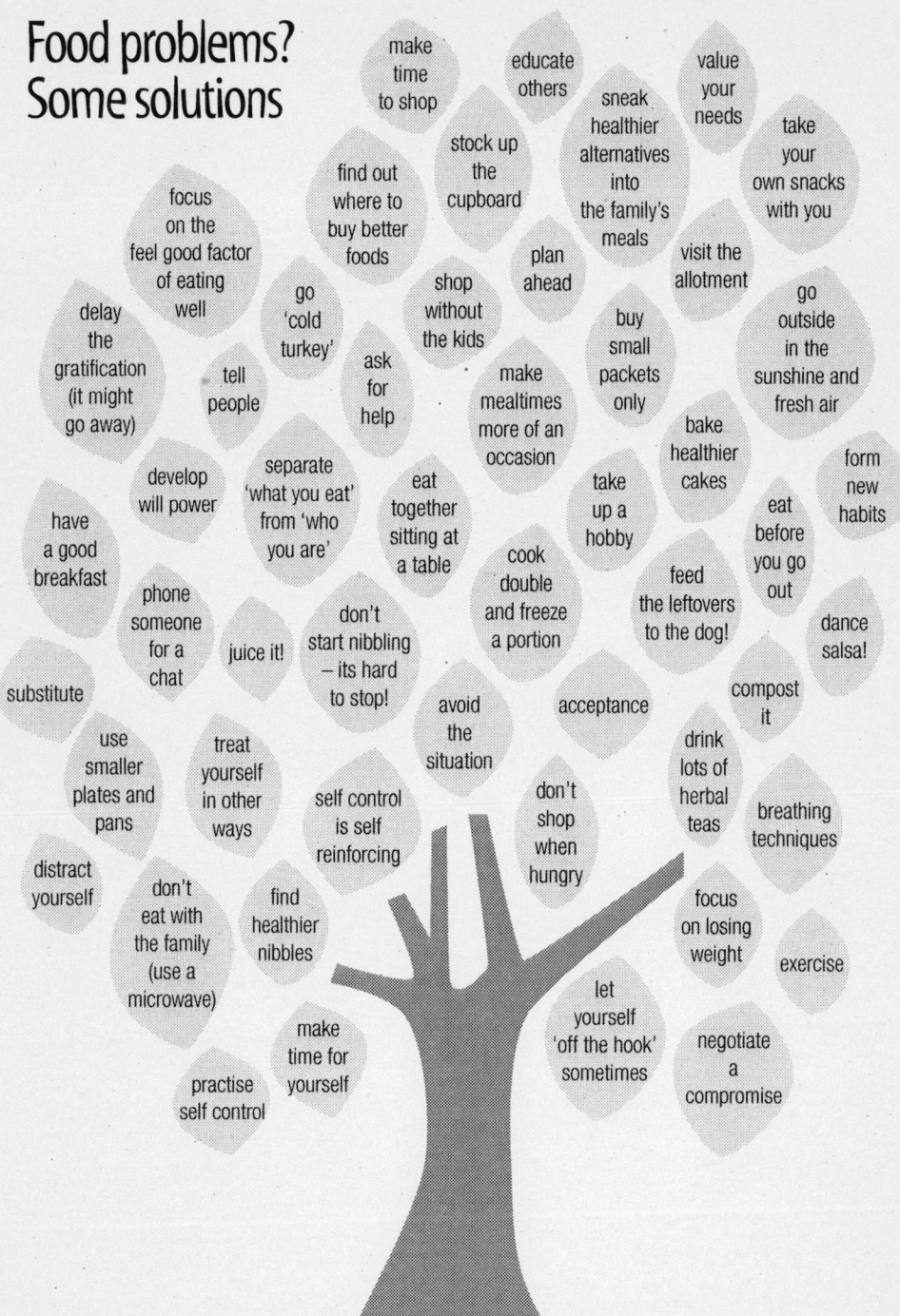

Food tasting

It is easier to change what you eat gradually, taking it one choice at a time. And remember that the next opportunity you have to change what you eat is the next time you put something into your mouth.

However, trying new things involves a financial risk of buying something you won't like. This risk is considerably reduced if it can be shared with others. As 'one person's meat can be another person's poison' it is likely that a group food tasting session with a selection of alternative foods to taste and drink will be able to provide something for everyone to take home with them.

The food tasting sessions were a popular part of the Food & Mood Project and the foods we tried were ready straight out of the packet. Here are some of the favourite alternatives the Food & Mood Project participants were able to try.

Milk alternatives
- Soya milk
  (remember to buy organic if you want to avoid GM foods)
- Rice Dream (plain or vanilla)
  (those sensitive to gluten need to be aware that this product contains barley proteins)
- Oat milk

Tea alternatives
- Hot water with a slice of lemon
- Cats claw
- Green tea
- Rooibosh (Red Bush) tea
- Peppermint herbal tea
- Camomile herbal tea
- Yogi tea
- Blackcurrant herbal tea
- Fennel herbal tea
- St John's wort herbal tea

Coffee alternatives
These are made from various grains including rye and barley plus chicory, figs and even acorns! They all taste different so keep sampling them until you find the one you like.

- Barley Cup
- Bambu
- Caro
- Dandelion Root
- Instant Chicory
- Nocaf
- Wake Up
- Yannoh

My food journey

My journey has been through vegetarianism, veganism (with fish!) and back to (organic) meat eating minus dairy, sugar and wheat products. Over the last year I thought I had Candida and went on a very restricted diet, but finally testing (a stool test) showed I had parasites. Fed up of popping supplements by the hundreds for a year, I began 'macrobiotic' food eating, but am not strict and now take Chinese herb supplements which have really helped.

I believe nutrition should come from food and it is too easy to 'pop pills' and now I want to look more at my diet and move towards a balanced, more macrobiotic food intake. My journey I feel has moved from western to eastern medicine and I think westerners are much more 'passive' and don't take responsibility for keeping healthy but reach for a quick-fix (pills) when they crack up. We can learn a lot from the care and attention a lot of eastern traditions take over food and health. I feel we need to be more actively responsible in our every day habits.

Rachel Austin
Food & Mood Project participant

Cold drinks alternatives
- Mineral water
- Carrot juice
- Beetroot juice
- Apple juice
- Prune juice
- Grape juice
- Orange juice
- 'Ame'
- 'Aqua Libra'

Juices can be diluted with water to reduce the sugar content of a drink and still taste sweet

Alternative quick-snacks
- Carob bar (a chocolate alternative)
- Flapjacks (these are usually wheat-free)
- Fruit 'strips' (pure fruit compressed into strips which can be sandwiched between oatcakes)
- Halva (a sweet tasting snack made from sesame seeds)
- Oat cakes
- Rice cakes
- Rice crackers
- Corn crackers
- Rye crackers
- Corn crisps
- Vegetable crisps
- Popcorn

Seeds, dried fruit and nuts
Delicious mixed with breakfast cereals or on their own as a snack.
- Sunflower seeds
- Pumpkin seeds
  These seeds are even better toasted and delicious sprinkled with soya or tamari (wheat free) sauce
- Dried figs
- Dried apricots
- Dried dates
- Cashew nuts
- Walnuts
- Almonds

Fruit & Veg
Fruit and some vegetables (such as carrots, celery, caulifower or red/green/yellow peppers) which can be eaten raw make excellent snacks. It is recommended that we eat *at least* five portions of fruit and vegetables every day – and this doesn't include potatoes!

The Food & Mood Project

We all came together
  from all walks of life
We came with our problems
  which were many and rife
We tried the alternatives
  with tasting and drinking
The info we got, gave us
  plenty of thinking
We studied the effects
  our mood had on eating
The allergies and cravings
  they all took a beating
We shared information
  and tried the new theories
We had a good laugh
  and related our stories
We read all the books
  and showed we all care
But the very best thing was
  It made us AWARE!

Diane Mitchell
Food & Mood Project
participant

Genetic engineering

Be aware: our staple diets – wheat, maize/corn, potatoes, tomatoes etc are in danger of yet further abuse (other than toxic sprays): genetic engineering.

Be aware: the long term outlook on genetic engineering is *unknown*.

If further information is required contact Genetix Snowball on 0161 834 0295.

Olive – Food & Mood Project participant

Taking supplements

Many psychological symptoms can be linked to nutritional deficiencies which, when treated with nutritional supplements, can be dramatically improved. Of course, taking supplements is no substitute for eating a varied and balanced diet containing plenty of fresh fruit and vegetables. However, regular supplementation can provide protection against deficiencies arising from erratic eating, illnesses which require additional nutritional support and the effects of environmental pollution. Supplements can also help to redress the imbalances caused by foods that contain artificial chemicals or which is of a poor nutritional quality.

Compared to the effort required in changing your diet, taking nutritional supplements has the advantage of involving the least disruption to daily life. Taking supplements and changing your diet at the same time is likely to achieve the greatest gains in the least amount of time but the disadvantage of doing several things at once is that you cannot be certain which change is having which benefit.

- Water is probably the most important cost effective 'nutrient' and has a profound effect on how we feel – aim for at least 8 glasses per day, preferably not tap water.

- If you can afford to take only one supplement, take a quality multi-mineral and vitamin supplement. This may be all you need to redress nutritional imbalances, correct faulty biochemistry and support the body's detoxification processes. A 'multi' also provides a firm foundation before 'topping up' with other nutrients, if and when these are needed.

- Buy the best supplements you can afford. If shopping around for a bargain and comparing products make sure you read the labels to compare the actual amounts of each nutrient. Bioavailability – how easily your body can absorb and use the nutrients – is an important consideration and generally worth paying for.

- Essential fats – particularly those found in oil-rich fish such as mackerel, salmon, sardines and tuna, and also in linseed/flax oil – are available in supplement form and are important to include if these foods are not eaten several times per week.

- Other beneficial nutrients include the B group vitamins and the minerals magnesium and zinc. (A simple zinc taste test taken by Food & Mood participants showed that over 90% were low in zinc).

- Overdosing on supplements is possible if you start to 'pick and mix' nutrients without reading further or asking professional advice. A leaflet 'The Safe Use of Supplements Benefits Good Health' available free from the Council for Responsible Nutrition, St Mary's Business Centre, Oystershell Lane, Newcastle upon Tyne, NE4 5QS, tel: 0191 232 3100 (send a large sae) provides useful information on agreed limits.

Further reading: Pfeiffer, C & Holford, P (1996) *Mental Health & Illness – the nutrition connection*, ION Press.

The Food & Mood Project library

Allergies

Anthony, H, Birtwistle, S, Eaton, K, Maberly, J (1997) *Environmental Medicine in Clinical Practice* BSAENM Publications, Southampton, UK.

Braly, J (1992) *Dr Braly's Food Allergy & Nutrition Revolution* Keats Publishing Inc, USA.

Brostoff, J & Gamlin, L (1989) *The Complete Guide to Food Allergy and Intolerance* Bloomsbury, London.

Carter, J & Edwars, A (1997) *The Rotation Diet Cookbook* Element Books Ltd.

Maberly, J & Anthony, H (1989) *Allergy : a practical guide to coping* The Crowood Press, Wiltshire, UK.

Mackarness, R (1976) *Not All In The Mind* Pan Books Ltd, London.

Philpott, W & Kalita, D (1980) *Brain Allergies: The Psycho Nutrient Connection* Keats Publishing Inc.

Reader's Digest (1998) *Fighting Allergies* Caroll and Brown Ltd, London

Mental Health

Barnes, B & I Colquhoun (1998) *Hyperactive Children* Thorsons.

DesMaisons, K (1998) *Potatoes Not Prozac* Simon & Schuster UK Ltd, London.

Hoffman, R (1997) *Attention Deficit Disorder* Keats Publishing Inc.

Holford, P (1995) *Mental Illness – not all in the mind* ION Press, London.

Lombard, J & Germano, C (1997) *The Brain Wellness Plan* Kensington Books, London.

Orbach, S (1993) Second Edition *Hunger Strike* Penguin Books, London.

Pfeiffer, C & Holford, P (1996) *Mental Health & Illness – the nutrition connection* ION Press, London.

Schauss, A (1997) *Anorexia & Bulimia* Keats Publishing Inc.

General

Schmidt, M (1997) *Smart Fats* Frog Ltd, USA.

Batmanghelidji, F (1992) *Your body's many cries for water* Redwood Books, UK.

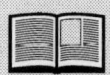

Review

Potatoes Not Prozac
Kathleen DesMaisons PhD
1998

This is a really good book, particularly if you think that you may be sensitive to sugar. It is easy to understand. She takes you by the hand through the different stages of her programme in an encouraging way. If you follow this programme you will achieve something, not only learning new information. She does explain some of the chemical effects of food – in an easy to understand way. Sugar sensitivity can affect physical and mental health. A positive book. Has a newsletter and web site (see page 236).

Reviewed by Julia

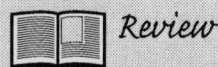

Review

Food & Healing
Annemarie Colbin 1986

Food & Healing is a mixture of Annemarie's personal theories/understanding of nutrition. She talks about foods and their energies. It is really good to think about what normally just gets shovelled into my mouth. She goes through different problems and possible solutions, different types of food (leaves, roots, dairy, etc) and what these can do for our bodies. She is into people taking responsibility for what they eat and thinks of it in physical, psychological and intellectual terms.

Reviewed by Julia

Colbin, A (1986) *Food & Healing* Ballantine Books, New York.

Elgin, D (1993) Revised edition *Voluntary Simplicity* Quill, William Morrow & Co.

Erasmus, U (1993) *Fats that Heal, Fats That Kill* Alive Books, Canada.

Holford, P (1997) *The Optimum Nutrition Bible* Piatkus, London.

Ledwards, C (1992) *Women, Food & Health* South Manchester Nutrition and Dietetic Service, UK. (This is a teaching pack).

Leeds, A, Brand Miller, J, Foster-Powell, K, Colagiuri, S (1996) *The GI Factor* Hodder & Stoughton, London.

Murray, M T & Pizzorno, J E (1990) *Encyclopaedia of Natural Medicine* Little, Brown & Company (UK), London.

Vegibake

(my favourite recipe)
This recipe is ideal for anyone with food sensitivities. it is wheat free, dairy free, sugar free, yeast free and gluten free. It is a very nutritious and filling dish which can be eaten on its own or with meat or poultry. It can also be served with an almond or cheese sauce (for those not allergic to dairy produce).
Serves 4 people.

4 carrots	2oz sunflower seeds
2 parsnips	2 tblspns olive oil
1/2 red onion	1 tspn dried herbs
1/2 lb broccoli	1lb potatoes
1/2 medium cauliflower	1/4 swede
1/2 frozen peas	1/2 turnip
4 tomatoes	salt, pepper to taste
4 tblspns water	

Grease a large roasting tin. Peel and cut all the vegetables – except the potatoes – into bite sized pieces. Pour the water into the roasting tin. Place all the mixed vegetables – except the potatoes – into the tin. Sprinkle the herbs, salt and pepper over the vegetables. Peel the potatoes and slice them, approx 1/4" wide. Dry the slices of potato on kitchen paper. Arrange the potatoes on top of the vegetables with each slice overlapping the next one. Pour the olive oil over the potatoes and sprinkle the sunflower seeds on top. Bake in preheated oven (mark 6) for approx 1 hour or until the potatoes are golden brown on top and soft inside.

Sylvia Hyland – Food & Mood Project participant

Food & mood
Some useful contacts

Organisations

Allergy Induced Autism (AIA)
3 Palmera Avenue, Calcot,
Reading, Berks RG3 7DZ
Tel: 0121 444 6450

Action Against Allergy
PO Box 278, Twickenham,
Middlesex, TW1 4QQ
Tel: 020 8892 2711

Action for ME
PO Box 1302,
Wells BA5 1YE
Tel: 01749 670799

Allergy Research Foundation
Middlesex Hospital
London W1N 8AA

Berrydales
Berrydale House
5 Lawn Road
London NW3 2XS
Tel: 0171 722 2866

British Allergy Foundation
Deepdene House
30 Bellegrove Road, Welling
Kent DA16 3YP
Tel: 0181 303 8525

British Association of
Nutritional Therapists (BANT)
BCM Bant
London WC1N 3XX
Tel: 0870 606 1284

British Society for Allergy
Environmental and Nutritional
Medicine (BSAENM)
PO Box 28, Totton
Southampton SO40 2ZA
Tel: 01703 812124

Eating Disorders Association (EDA)
Sackville Place
44 Magdalene Street
Norwich, Norfolk NR3 1IU
Tel: 01603 619 090 (admin)
Tel: 01603 621 414 (helpline)

The Hyperactive Childrens
Support Group (HACSG)
71 Wyke Lane, Chichester
East Sussex PO19 2LD
Tel: 01903 725182

The Society for the Promotion
of Nutritional Therapy (SPNT)
PO Box 626
Woking GU22 OXD
Tel: 01483 740903

ME Association
4 Corringham Road
Stamford le Hope
Essex SS17 AOH
Tel: 01375 642 466

Mind
Granta House
15-19 Broadway, Stratford
London E15 4BQ
Tel: 0181 519 2122

Allergy Testing

York Nutritional Laboratory
Lysander Close, Clifton Moor
York YO30 4XB
Tel: 01904 690640

Alternative Food Sources

AllergyCare
1 Church Square, Taunton
Somerset TA1 1SA
Tel: 01823 325023

Allergyfree Direct Ltd
5 CentreMead
Osney Mead OX2 0ES
Tel: 01865 722003

Berrydales
Berrydale House
5 Lawn Road
London NW3 2XS
Tel: 0171 722 2866

Pure Organics Ltd
Stockport Farm
Stockport Road, Amesbury
Wilts SP4 7LN
0800 783 7535

Nutritional Supplements
(quality nutritional supplements mail order)

BioCare
Lakeside, 180 Lifford Lane,
Kings Norton
Birmingham B30 3NT
Tel: 0120 433 3727

Higher Nature
Burwash Common
East Sussex TN19 7LX
Tel: 01435 883844

Lamberts
1 Lambert Road
Tunbridge Wells
Kent TN2 3EQ
Tel: 01892 552120

Clinics

Airedale Allergy Centre
High Hall, Steeton, Keighley
West Yorkshire BD20 6SB
Tel: 01535 603966

Breakspear Hospital
Lord Alexander House
Waterhouse Street
Hemel Hempstead
Herts HP1 1DL
Tel: 01442 261333

The Children's Clinic at Dolphin
House
(registered charity providing
complementary therapies for
children)
14 New Road, Brighton
East Sussex BN1 1UF
Tel: 01273 324790

Feedback!

If you are able to try any of the suggestions in this Workbook, The Food & Mood Project is compiling a record of people's experiences.

Please write telling us of the changes you made and the benefits to your health and your life to:

The Food & Mood Project
PO Box 2737
LEWES
East Sussex BN7 2GN
UK

We look forward to hearing from you.